# SNAKEBITE!

## Marjory Wildcraft

**grow**network™

www.TheGrowNetwork.com

**SNAKEBITE!** *How I Successfully Treated a Venomous Snakebite at Home:*
*The 5 Essential Preparations You Need to Have*

by Marjory Wildcraft

ISBN: 978-0-9995663-0-5

**grow**network™

www.TheGrowNetwork.com
PO Box 415
Red Rock, TX  78662
United States
(877) 799 3878

http://thegrownetwork.com

# SNAKEBITE!

## How I Successfully Treated a Venomous Snakebite at Home

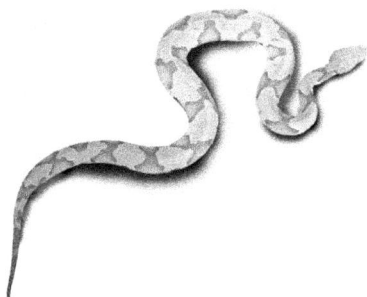

## The 5 Essential Preparations You Need to Have

# Marjory Wildcraft

# Contents

# Acknowledgments

First and foremost, I thank my family—my husband David, and my kids Ryan and Kimber.  As you read this little book, you'll see how much I love and depend on them.

There are many fine herbalists that I have learned from, and I would especially like to thank Doug Simons and Nicole Telkes.

This book would not have been possible without the help of Carol Hiltner whose editing, layout, and design skills brought this book into reality.  I also want to thank Michael Ford who did the initial editing.

And finally, I want to thank the entire Grow Network team: Sharon Porter, Anthony Tamayo, Jimerson Adkins, Jennifer Boulet, Merin Porter, and Nikki Follis. It is so much fun to work with you!

# I Was Breaking the No. 1 Rule in Homesteading and in Life

The No. 1 rule in homesteading and life is:

> *Never put your hands or feet where you can't see them.*

That's such a great rule, and it will keep you safe on your homestead as well as throughout life in general.

I was barefoot on my way to the tomato patch. I hadn't wanted this jungle of indeterminate tomato plants. But a freeze had wiped out my initial planting of the more orderly bushes of paste tomatoes.

(If you don't know what indeterminate tomatoes are, or you would like to see some video of the tomato patch, check out this short video: http://thegrownetwork.com/homesteading-basics-determinate-vs-indeterminate-tomatoes/#comment-19576.)

These unwanted tomato plants had megalomaniacal tendencies. They created a forest that sprawled and climbed all over everything. They were producing way more foliage than tomatoes. So I had to plunge deep into the patch to find anything.

# A Blessing and a Curse

But wow, did I start grinning when my explorations revealed a fat, 6-inch diameter beefsteak tomato hanging in the shade.

My mouth started to water as I cradled the heavy beauty.

Whew, I had no idea this thing had been growing in there. Oh, the bragging rights! It is almost impossible to grow this big beautiful variety in our climate. And this was a showcase specimen. Were there any more?

Pushing further into the nightshade jungle, I felt a cat's claw vine hook into the top of my foot. Reactively jerking my foot, I felt the barb work its way in deeper.

*Ouch!*

# That Wasn't a Cat's Claw

On second thought, I realized that there was a bigger problem.

There are no cat's claw vines, or any other plants with thorns, in my garden.

Hmm, was the sting from a really big scorpion?

Actually it felt sort of like an ice pick in the top of my foot. It was stronger than a spider bite for sure. And it definitely hurt more than fire ants.

## What could it be?

Brushing aside the tangle of tomato plant branches, I knelt down. I saw two neat puncture wounds in the top of my left foot and one big drop of blood. The three of them made a perfect equilateral triangle with about ¼" sides.

# Snake Bite!

The first rule of snake encounters is:

*Stay calm.*

Okay, so I needed to stay calm.

I took a deep breath and went through the snakebite facts I knew.

The CDC (American Center for Disease Control and Prevention) states that venomous snakes bite only 7,000 to 8,000 people in the US each year. And only about 5 of these people die. (http://www.cdc.gov/niosh/topics/snakes/)

I didn't really know those exact specifics at the moment, but I did know it was something like that. Anyway, I figured the odds were in my favor and it helped to keep me calm.

# Identifying the Culprit

The second rule of snakebites is:

*Try to identify the snake.*

You don't want to spend a ton of time doing this.

Ideally, you should know the snakes that live in your area ahead of time. Be familiar with what they look like so you can identify them quickly.

"Hopefully it was just a rat snake, or a king snake," I thought. We have a lot of those guys, as they like to eat my chickens' eggs. They also do valuable work eating mice and rodents in the barn so I don't get too upset at them being around.

Plus, rat and king snakes aren't venomous. If one of them bites you, the worst thing that can happen is the wound getting infected. And preventing infection is easy with good wound care.

So I would be happy if it were a rat or king snake bite.

Delighted, really, when you consider the other options.

# Using the Process of Elimination

The snake with the deadliest venom in my area is the coral snake with its bright red, yellow, and black bands. They look sort of like a corn snake, which is also occasionally in this area. The way to tell the difference between the two is to remember that famous poem:

> *Red next to yellow, kill a fellow,*
> *red next to black, okay for Jack.*

I do see the deadly coral snakes from time to time, but they are always very small. In fact, their mouths are generally too small to do much of anything to humans—except if they get a small toe or finger. But it is extremely rare in my area to get bitten—or die—from a coral snake.

Plus, the way this bite was on top of my foot I knew it couldn't be a coral snake.

But I looked around under the tomato plants for the bright colors anyway, just in case. Even though I know all of this, a sigh of relief slipped out when didn't see a coral snake anywhere.

I continued looking for any kind of snake.

# Know Your Local Snakes

The rattlesnake, for which the Southwest is famous, can certainly kill you. Or at least make your life miserable for many weeks! According to *Wikipedia*, of the 20 venomous snakes in the US, 16 of them are some form of rattlesnake.

But rattlers prefer rocky outcroppings and I have never seen a rattlesnake on our sandy, post oak savannah land. None of my closest neighbors had ever seen a rattler either.

*How do you know what kind of snakes live in your area?*

Especially if have just moved in? Here are three suggestions:

- Start asking the neighbors. Everyone has snake stories. (You may hear more than you want, but at least you'll know what can be around.)

- Your local extension office, which probably has a wildlife biologist on staff, will also know.

- And finally, one of my favorite go-to wildlife books is the *Readers Digest Guide to North*

*American Wildlife* available here at Amazon: http://astore.amazon.com/wwwbackyardfo-20/detail/1606524917 (Yes, yes, The Grow Network earns like 15 cents if you buy it through this link). This book is for all of North America, and there are lots of great books out there for your region. Look around and I am sure you'll find one.

- And, since the Grow Network is a global community, I dug through the Internet and sourced some other free resources to help you. Below are some good online PDF docs with photos and identification guides for snakes.

Hey, if you know of a good resource for identifying snakes in your area, why not drop me a line at happiness@thegrownetwork.com. I would love to hear from you.

- South African venomous snakes (28-page document with 10 extremely deadly snakes in that region... including the Black Mamba. Nice photos and detailed descriptions): http://www.hikinginfo.co.za/DOCS/Snake Guide.pdf

- Venomous Snakes of Nepal (86-page document with beautiful photos covering kraits, cobras, king cobras, coral snakes, vipers, and pit vipers): http://www.bik-f.de/files/publications/kuch_venomous_snakes_of_nepal_-_english_edition.pdf

- SNAKES: Pictorial Key To Venomous Species In United States (4-page document with very detailed line drawings of snake heads and how to identify venomous snakes): http://www.cdc.gov/nceh/ehs/Docs/Pictorial_Keys/Snakes.pdf

The main takeaway from all this is:

*It is important to be familiar with the snakes that share your neighborhood.*

# The Last Option: Copperhead

So I was pretty sure it wasn't a coral snake or a rattler. The other options were some of our more harmless snakes...or the final concern—a copperhead.

I knew that while a copperhead bite could also be a very painful experience—sometimes dragging on for weeks—it is rarely fatal.

Since I didn't see any snakes around, and I didn't want to spend a ton of time looking for the snake (and you shouldn't either) I walked back to the house.

My husband Dave was in the kitchen.

"I've been snake-bit."

"Do you know what kind?" he asked.

"No."

He came over and looked at my foot. The drop of blood had smeared into a big Nike swoosh. He glanced up at the clock. "It's about 7:45, did it just happen?"

"Yes."

"Does it hurt?"

"It is starting to," I said.

## "Copperhead, then."

He looked again. "Hmm, punctures about $^1/_4$" to $^3/_8$" apart....It was a young'un."

We both had heard the stories that baby copperheads are more dangerous because they can't control their venom and they inject all they have. I don't know if that theory is true or not. And I guessed that while young, this one wasn't a baby.

But it is true that the venom in a young snake is just as dangerous as in a fully-grown adult. The feeling of the fangs digging in when I jerked my foot back haunted me. I had probably gotten a good-sized dose.

# Herbal Care for Snake Bites

"What should we poultice it with?" Dave asked.

Being late June, I had no cabbages on hand. The plantain plants that grow on our land are very narrow leafed and tiny. It would take forever to gather enough.

I racked my brain. I thought of the half-gallon jar of dried nettle leaf on the shelf in the pantry. But it wouldn't be enough, and I wasn't sure that was a good poultice material anyway.

*"Prickly pear pads," I said.*

"The ones behind the cow shed are a thornless variety and good sized."

There really is no such thing as a thornless prickly pear, but some are less thorny than others.

Years ago there had been a Craigslist ad for free thornless cactus plants that needed to be rescued or they would be destroyed. A girlfriend and I made the expedition into Austin and filled up two big sacks full of the pads. I planted them behind the cowshed where it tends to be very hot and dry, which is what they like. I occasionally cut back the grass from around them, but they mostly thrived in their new home with little help from me. Over the years they have given me much medicine and food.

Actually, if you want to see the patch, it is the same one in which we filmed Doug Simons harvesting pads to use in the video we created on treating infections without antibiotics: http://try.thegrownetwork.com/tiwa/.

# Our Living Room Rug: Workshop, Community Center, Hospital, and More...

> *"I am going to take a cold shower to reduce my blood circulation and I'll be lying down here in the living room when you get back."*

I pointed to the big rug. Everything of importance in our family happens either around the dining table or on the living room rug.

Every evening my family gathers around the rug to hang out together. Through the years, most of my kid's school projects were created on the living room rug. Vast amounts of artwork have been created on the rug. Countless wrestling matches, yoga sessions, and gymnastics events have been held on the rug. At Christmas, the wrappings from piles of presents will be ripped open on the rug. I birthed my daughter on the living room rug.

No, it is not the same rug through the decades. With all that activity we change the rug out every few years.

# I'm Not Afraid to Break the Rules...a Little

Technically, by the rules, I should have lain down immediately and skipped the cold shower. But I was hot and dirty from outdoor work and I correctly guessed that things were going to get much worse. I didn't want to go into this experience sticky and smelly.

The third rule of snakebites is:

*Lie down as soon as possible.*

Dave took a long time to get the prickly pear pads. By the time he got back my foot had swollen enough that you could no longer see the puncture marks. And the pain was increasing.

It was definitely a copperhead bite.

# Poulticing a Snake Bite with Prickly Pear

Dave had made poultices of cabbage for me years ago when I had mastitis.

*But he had never harvested prickly pear, nor made a poultice from it before.*

He knew the general principles as he had seen me treat myself for other injuries. He is not the kind of guy to ask for, or read, directions. So he went at it boldly on his own.

He decided to skin the outside of a big pad and scar it crisscross with a knife to give it some flexibility. He attempted to apply this to my foot by tying it together with some cloth strips I keep in the medical bag.

I wondered if this technique might actually work.

It didn't.

Dave sort of understood it wasn't right and asked, "Is this okay?"

You certainly don't want to upset the people who are helping you in an emergency. I said, "Hon, I realize now why Doug always takes apart the pad to make a slimy mush for the poultice. That way the material can fit to the contour of the body. The one you made doesn't get that much good contact."

He nodded with understanding while trying to work a small thorn out of his finger.

I mentioned:

"If you take two big rocks, you can use them to scrape all the thorns off the pad before you remove the pad from the plant. It makes it super easy to harvest."

# Warding Off Infection after a Snake Bite

As he headed back out to the prickly pear patch to get more to try again, I asked my 15-year-old daughter Kimber to prepare me some garlic. She peeled a fresh clove and crushed it with the side of a knife. Then she minced it. She brought me a tablespoon of the garlic mash medicine and a small glass of water as a chaser.

*I wanted the garlic for insurance against internal infection.*

I was about to ask her for some echinacea tincture when a wave of pain came.

*Echinacea would have been good to help my immune system.*

But as events unfolded, I never got around to asking for it and it was forgotten.

If you would like a free, easy-to-read report I wrote on how to use garlic as your first home medicine, just go to http://garlicmiracle.com.

# Here Comes the Pain

Pain tends to come in waves, and it was rising much like an incoming ocean tide. Coming in strongly, backing off a bit, and then surging to a new level of intensity.

With the next low in pain, I started giving Kimber directions on how to log into my account in the Grow Network's Honors Lab (a site for backyard researchers to share, learn, and create resources for sustainable living) and where to find the video on treating snakebites.

Dave came back from the prickly pear patch more quickly this time.

*"How's the pain?" he asked.*

We all laughed for a moment at the absurdity of that question.

Dave remembered the thing paramedics and doctors always ask: "On a scale of 1 to 10, how much pain are you feeling right now?"

That seemed funny, too. But we decided that a 1 or 2 was your typical fire ant bites or small scratches that drew some blood. Level 10 was so bad you were on the precipice of passing out. At about 5 or 6 the pain demanded most of your attention, but was manageable.

I decided it was going in waves between a level 3 and 7. At its peaks, the pain absolutely demanded my full attention, but I had certainly endured worse.

Dave nodded agreement with my assessment. A copperhead had bitten him just three years before, so he knew what I was going through.

# When Poulticing a Snakebite... GO BIG!

Things started getting a little hazy for me as the waves came with more pain and less relief. I heard the sounds of chopping in the kitchen and the video going in the office.

Dave got a new slushier version of a poultice on my foot. It felt so good....The cool, slimy, green, soothing cactus was a good, good thing.

But there are two things about a poultice that most people get wrong.

> *The first mistake is that most people make poultices too small.*

You really need to cover a large area.

When I surfaced from the next round of pain, I told Dave, "You know what, Hon? We are going to need about four to five times more material. My whole foot needs to be encased in poultice."

Dave went back to the patch again and got more pads. He came back much faster this time and made a bigger poultice.

At some point I was vaguely surprised to become aware that both he and Kimber were in the office intently watching the Treating Infections without Antibiotics http://try.thegrownetwork.com/tiwa/ video and figuring out what to do.

Dave discovered that he could use the blender to speed up the process of making the prickly pear slurry.

He also figured out the following system for applying the poultice to this unusually-shaped area.

1. First he put my foot into an old pillowcase. He poured the prickly pear slurry in so it was covering and surrounding my foot.

2. Then he used a plastic bag to contain the oozing that was coming out of the pillowcase.

3. And finally, he wrapped the whole thing up with a towel and tied it in place with cloth strips.

*The second mistake is they don't keep the poultice on long enough.*

You need to keep it on for hours, overnight.

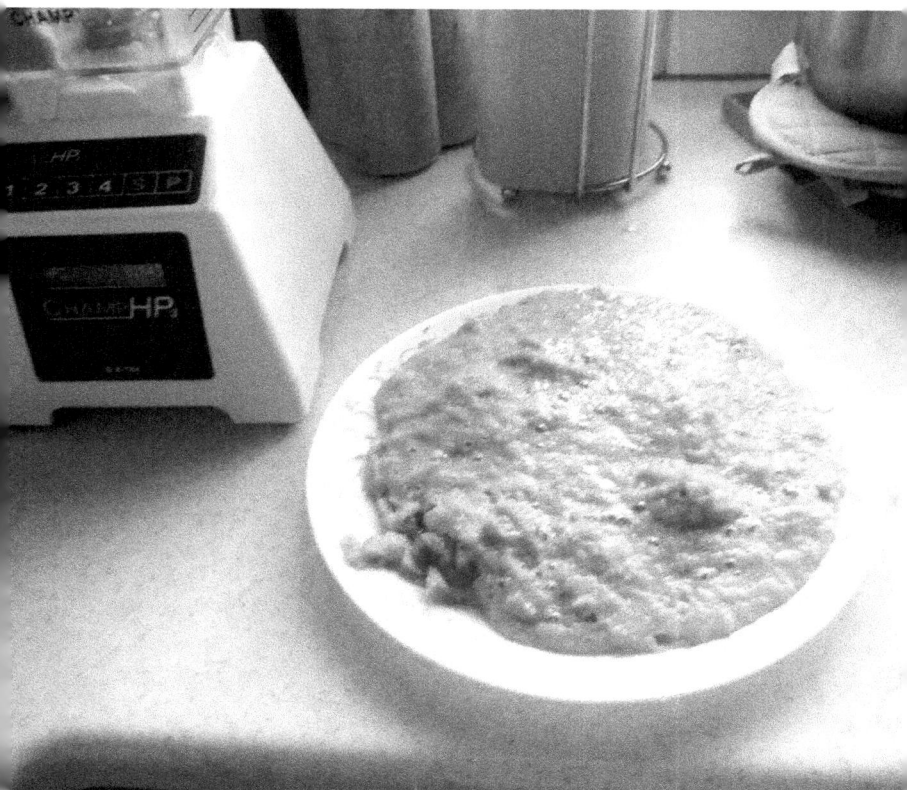

Dave figured out that a blender was the best way
to make the prickly pear slurry.

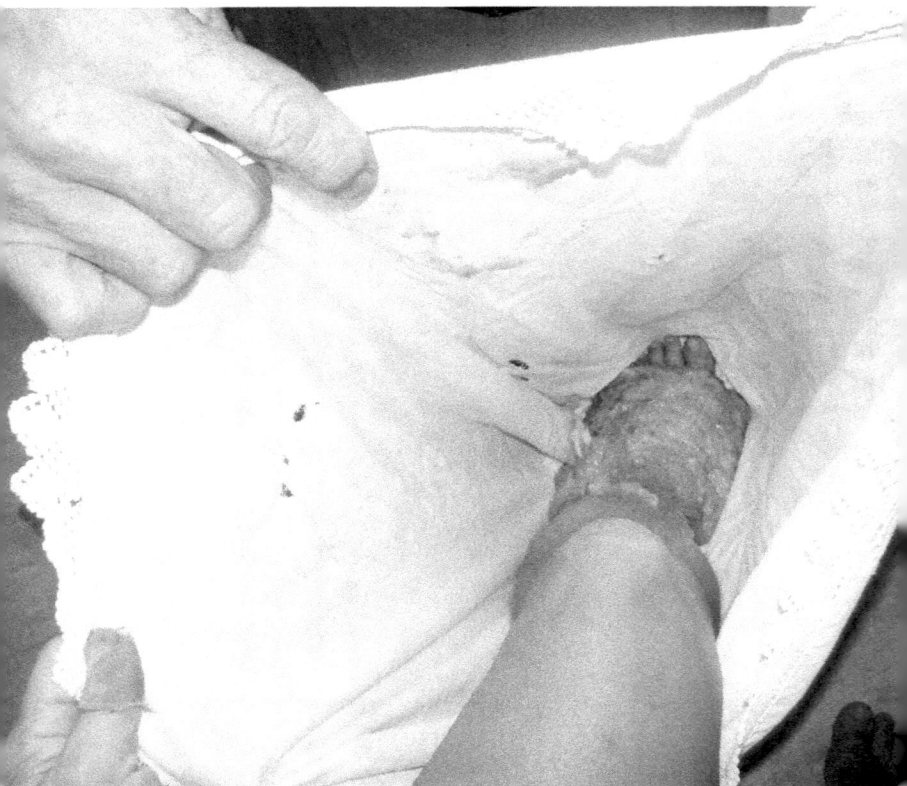

We poured the slurry into an old pillowcase
with my foot inside.

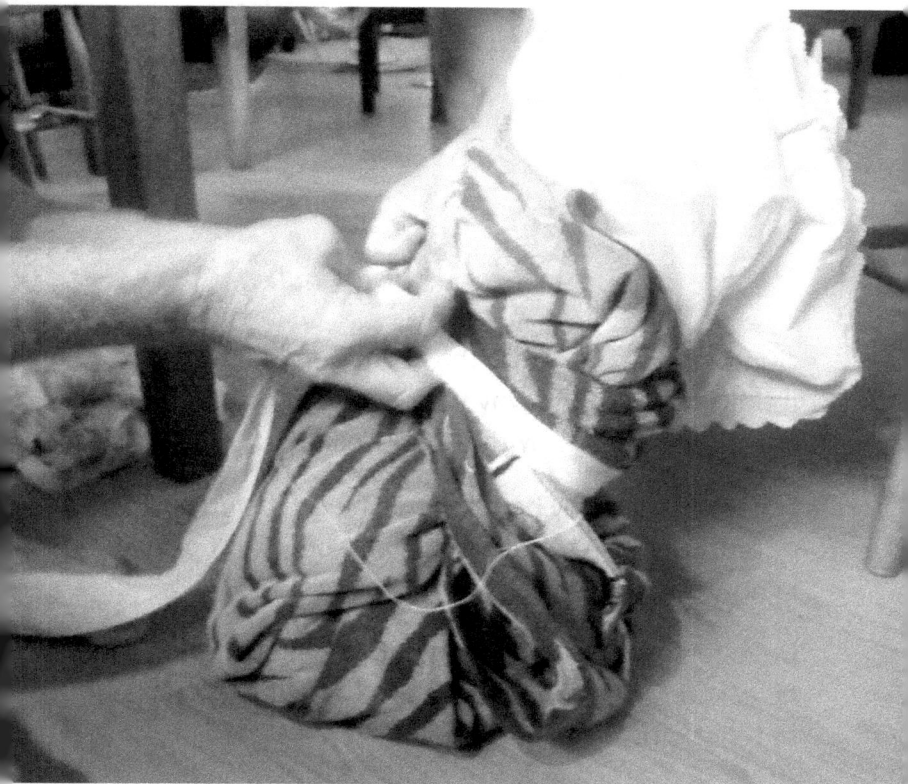

Tying the final bundle together

# Desperate Times Call for Desperate Measures

## The pain was increasing.

"Kimber, please get me that homemade pain medicine. It's in the way back of the pantry. The black stuff in the pint jar with the white lid."

Normally, all of my home medicine is labeled and dated. But this stuff is special and only Kimber and I know about it.

Dave furrowed his brow, "What is that stuff, Hon?" he asked. "If I end up taking you to the hospital I need to tell them...."

"It's a low grade level of morphine," I said. "It's nothing like the strong stuff they shot you up with."

Dave had been in such pain in the hospital when he was bitten.

*My homemade analgesic could take the edge off the pain—make it bearable.*

It wasn't strong enough to take all the pain away. But just taking the edge off is a really good thing sometimes.

I rarely used it, and when I did it was because I really needed it. It is pretty easy to grow the plants for it in your garden and process the medicine at home. I make a batch every few years so I always have a small supply on hand. (If you want to know the process, check out the article in the "Inside Edition," which is the private blog for those with <u>Honors Lab</u> access, but your local herbalist could probably teach you how to do it, too.)

Kimber got me an ounce or so of the medicine.

I now was mostly focused on dealing with pain that was swinging more from 5 to 8 on "the scale."

It was going to get much worse before the night was through. But every cloud has a silver lining, and in the coming agony I would have a deeply life-changing mystical experience.

# The Intense Pain
## of a Copperhead Bite

The pain was becoming loud, and it was filling up the room and bouncing off the walls. I began writhing on the living room rug. I sprawled this way and that, pinned down invisibly by my snake bitten left foot.

*I was groaning.*

For a brief moment Dave's face loomed over me. His mouth was set in a line and his eyes studied me, searching for something.

I heard him rush back to the office where my daughter was still watching the video. I could hear their voices, my daughter Kimber, occasionally Dave, and mostly Doug Simons as he explained in the video how traditional medicine worked. Their sounds came to me mixed in with the loudness of the pain.

I couldn't understand what they were saying.

I didn't care.

# Following Familiar Guidance

*Suddenly, in the middle of the pain and the roaring in my ears, I felt a quiet calm presence that joined with me.*

This presence was I, but not I. She was someone very familiar, very wise.

She pointed out that since I was writhing on the floor, why didn't I just go with it and proactively stretch my body?

I hadn't been to yoga in a few weeks and I was pretty stiff.

It seemed like a good idea.

*So I started to stretch and move my body ahead of the pain.*

I stretched like I do on glorious, lazy Sunday mornings when I just take up the whole bed and twist and reach and move everything.

It felt good.

Really good.

# Stretching with the Pain

*As long as I kept it up, there was only the familiar release of muscles stretching.*

Pain yes, but a familiar pain, an easy pain.

A good pain.

She calmly explained that new elements of reality would come with this venom, and I needed to be flexible.

When I say she "explained"—it wasn't like I was hearing any words. Or seeing visions of anyone. I just had a strong sense that this was true. And the words I am writing are my best attempt to explain what I understood at the time.

# My Surprise Spiritual Experience

Many spiritual traditions and mystery schools have a name for this kind of encounter: your higher self, guardian angel, or spirit guide are a few commonly used names.

I didn't see anyone, or hear any words.

*I just "knew" things that are not a normal part of what I know.*

I suppose you should always have some caution when dealing with this other layer of reality, as other beings may not necessarily have your best interests in mind.

But the suggestion to stretch had been a good one.

To an external observer, it may have appeared that I was flailing about on the floor. But internally, I was doing some really aggressive stretching.

Whatever. It was a good thing.

# The Purging Begins

*I did this for a time and
then I felt my gut start to tremble.*

The calm presence let me know that my body could not afford to waste any resources on digesting the food I had eaten earlier and it would have to go.

"Kimber, will you get me a big bowl please?"

She brought the big stainless steel bowl from the kitchen. I got up on my left elbow, leaned over the bowl, and retched.

*The calm presence told me
to breathe deeply.*

I hadn't realized that, while I was vomiting, I was holding my breath.

I breathed deeply through my nose down to my root and was surprised to find how much more easily the contents of my stomach came up.

For a moment, I forgot again to breath, tightening involuntarily and the retching was a painful struggle again.

"Breathe," the calm presence reminded me.

*I did, and again it felt miraculously easier.*

In my life I've had a few episodes of vomiting for one reason or another. And while this time wasn't exactly pleasant, it was the easiest time I've ever had of it.

I rested for a while, surprised at this new insight.

Kimber took the bowl away, emptied it somewhere, and brought it back rinsed clean.

I went through two more long rounds of vomiting.

# Accepting Change and Respecting the Snake

There was a pause here where I connected with the calm presence. I'll write it as best as I understand it, but again, it was not communicated in words or images. Just through direct understanding.

> *She told me that the venom of a snake is an important gift.*

If honored properly, it would mean big changes in my life. Most people are afraid of major changes, and that is the underlying cause of the deep fear many people have around snakes.

Unfortunately, she didn't have any specifics on just what changes would occur or exactly how I should honor the venom (although that would come later). I suppose the vagueness of the message is the problem with these kinds of encounters. But it was very reassuring and it helped me to relax into this whole process.

I had to agree with her that snakes have a really bad reputation that is largely undeserved. Adam and Eve immediately spring to mind whenever anyone says "snake." And that story didn't exactly have a happy ending.

# The Purging Continues

Physical reality came rushing back in with a new rudeness.

> *I discovered the contents of my colon had liquefied and needed to be released immediately.*

It came out violently. Dave barely got me to the bathroom in time.

The convulsions for this release also came in waves over a period of time. The calm presence told me that this, too, was simply a part of the process.

Like the contents of my stomach, what was in my bowels had to be gotten rid of. My body needed to focus resources on healing and not on processing waste.

When this part was finished, it was well into the night. Dave helped me to bed. I lay down with the poultice sloshing around my foot and a pillow under my knee. The pain was just a throb down there—a very manageable 1 or 2 on the pain scale.

My body was empty. Completely drained.

# The Deepest Breathing and the Slightest Stretch

I felt the calm presence again.

> *I understood that the way to honor the venom was to re-learn to breathe deeply as an everyday, "all the time" thing.*

Yes, yes, everyone takes a deep breath when they are stressed, and it is almost a joke to tell someone to take a deep breath when a situation starts to get out of hand. But seriously, if I would take on the challenge of actually breathing deeply as part of every moment of my life, many good changes would come.

She suggested I wear a bracelet. Every time I saw or touched the bracelet I should remind myself to breathe deeply. The bracelet could be of any material; it could be plain or colorful, simple or ornate, a gift or purchased. It didn't really matter. The bracelet's primary function was to trigger a reminder to breathe deeply.

And in the mornings for a few minutes before I get out of bed, I should stretch like I had earlier that night. Nothing too crazy. It could be done gently enough not to waken Dave if he were sleeping next to me. Just a few minutes' worth would be beneficial. Like a cat awakening from sleep.

Both of these suggestions made a lot of sense to me. Practical and simple, yet, I could see that there would be profound benefits. I promised myself, and "her"(?) that I would do these things and work to make them habitual.

Soon after that I was fast asleep.

# The Morning after My Venomous Snake Bite

I awoke late the next morning—my foot swollen and my mouth very dry.

Dave got me some water and I gingerly began to drink. We opened up the wrapping on my foot, wondering what my foot would look like. Dave joked that the prickly pear had slow-cooked through the night and smelled delicious.

It actually did smell good, and I am not sure he was completely joking.

*Overall, the swelling was slowly going down.*

He applied a fresh poultice to my foot, with new wrappings.

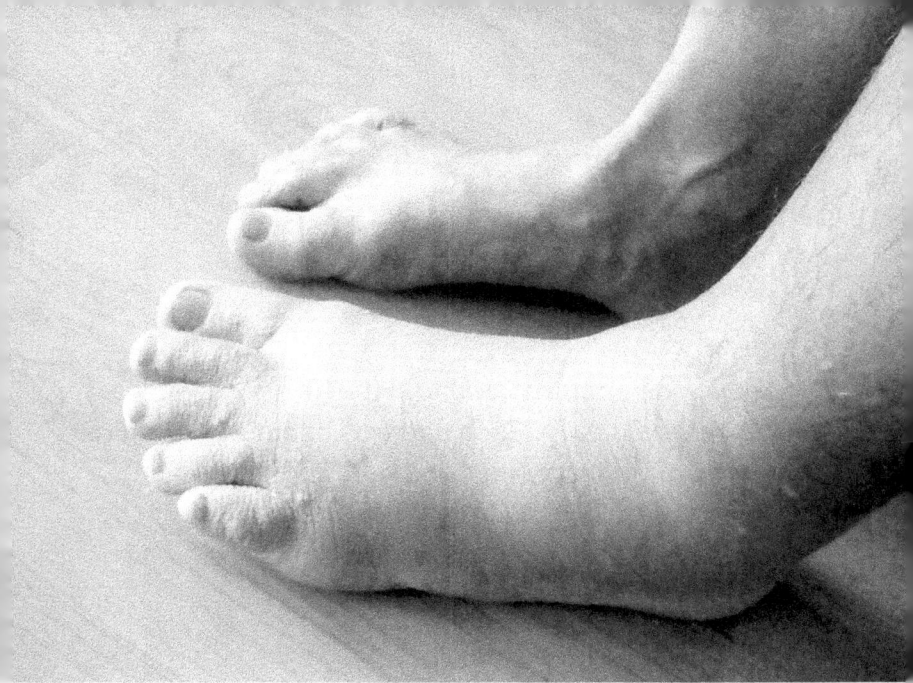

Snake bite—comparison of swollen foot to regular foot the first morning after poulticing

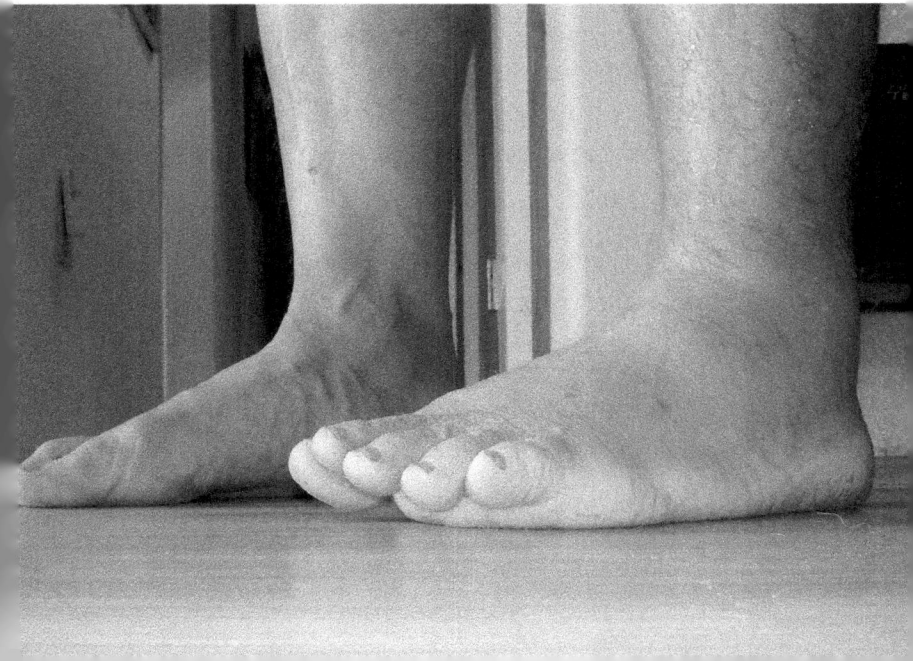

# Reapplying the Poultice and Follow-Up Care

To make one poultice Dave told me he needed at least two big cactus pads. Each pad was about 10" or more in diameter and about $^3/_4$" thick. Prickly pear cactus grows almost everywhere on Earth, so you should be able to have a patch if you want to grow your own.

*I slept a lot that day.*

I wasn't that hungry and I ate sparingly. To help rehydrate, I drank a lot of water, herbal teas, and some green juices.

The pair of crutches we keep by the medical kit came in very handy. I hobbled over to the office and did a bit of work on the computer. But mostly I stayed in bed, reading and sleeping.

There was no more vomiting, diarrhea, or even that much pain. My foot was swollen and tender, but there really wasn't much to say about it.

We kept the foot poulticed the entire day, changing it twice during the day and once more before I went to bed for the night.

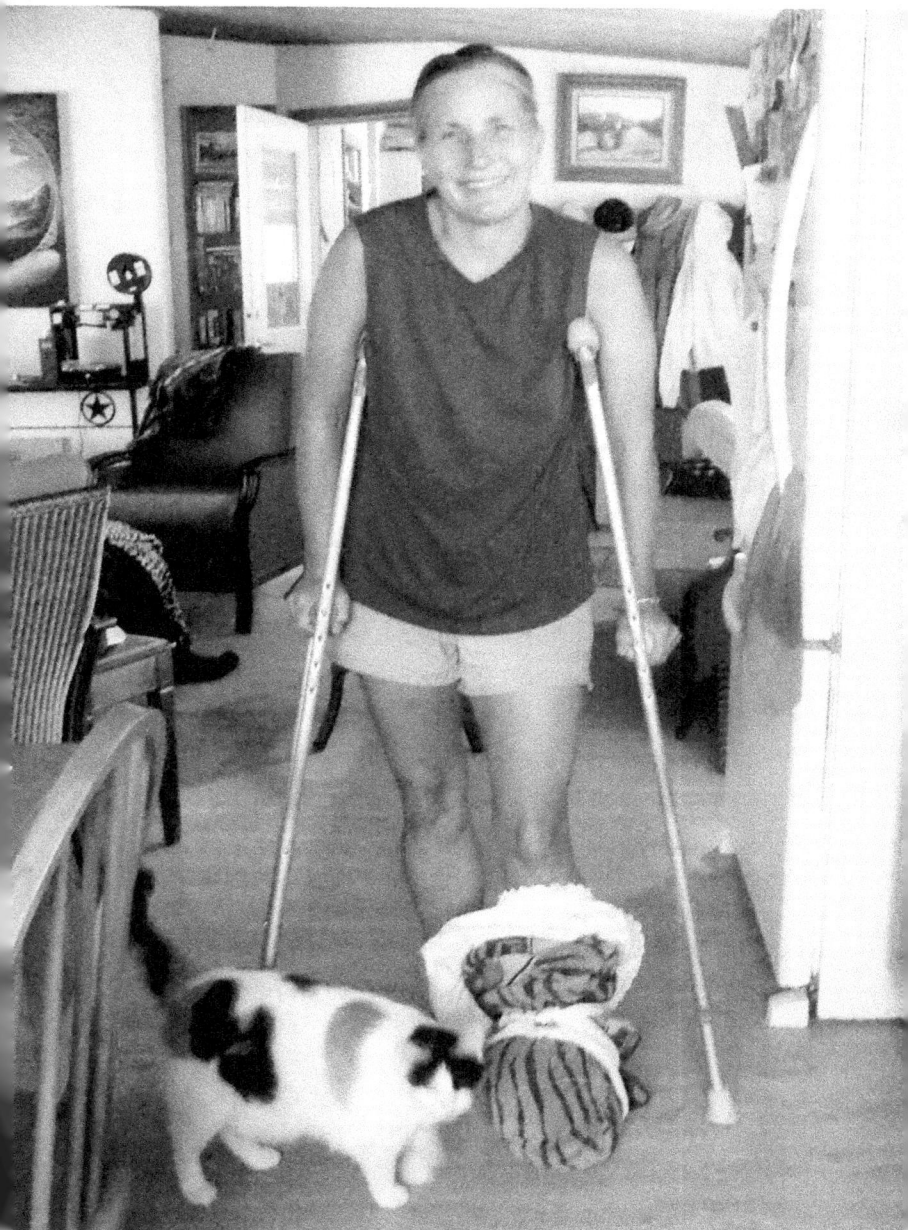

# The Second Morning— Sweet Relief

*The following morning I felt much better.*

We took the poultice off for a few hours and I could walk with only a bit of stiffness. I had Kimber drive the riding lawn mower over to the house and I used that to get around and do my chores.

We had a project where we were growing out 120 chickens for meat. These chickens were not the usual heritage breeds I normally work with, but Cornish rock crosses. "Franken birds"—they were somewhat unnatural creatures and I was having to really adjust my systems to accommodate them. We had been having some unusual die offs, which I think were due to the heat. But regardless, I was worried about them, and I was glad to be getting back to work.

I came back to the house and we poulticed my foot for the day. But other than a few extra naps I was mostly back to my normal life.

We had intended to poultice the foot that night, but I never got around to it. And by the following morning, other than a bit of residual swelling and some tenderness, I was essentially as good as usual.

The foot was only slightly swollen. I had a meeting in Austin, and the swelling was down so that I comfortably wore a pair of shoes that were normally a bit big for me.

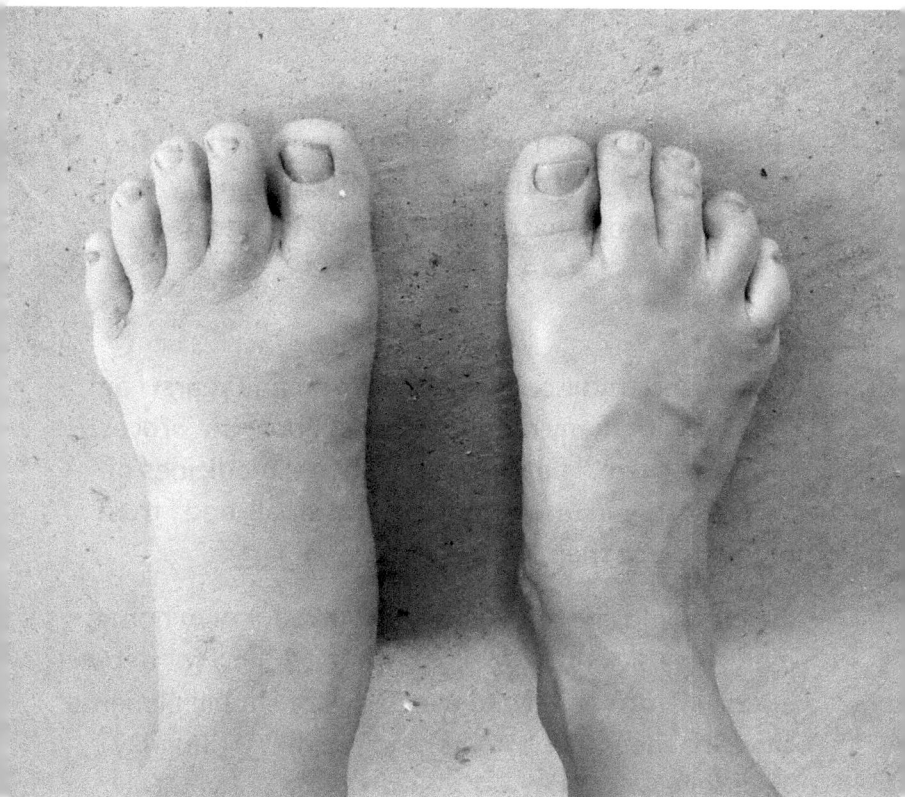

*Snake bite—second morning after swelling goes down*

# Looking Back on My Snake Bite Experience: The 5 Key Preparations

What factors went into this being a story with a happy ending? I think five key things were in place.

## 1.

I prepared ahead of time by being familiar with the snakes of my area and their potential for injury. And I had a plan for what to do in case of being bitten.

## 2.

I have used traditional medicine for many years. I am familiar with many medicines and I know the process for using them. I have used traditional medicines on several other injuries, both big and small, and I trust myself to use them well.

(If you would like to get started with your own home medicine, click on https://garlicmiracle.com/ for a free eBook I wrote on how to use garlic for simple ailments like ear aches, sore throats, and preventing holiday illnesses).

### 3.

I have a good sense of knowing what I can handle and when I should call for outside help (as in going to the hospital). And yes, knowing that there is the medical system as a backup plan is reassuring.

### 4.

I have a strong immune system from years of eating good food, exercising, and taking care of myself. I trust my body to heal.

### 5.

Most importantly, my family is very supportive and was willing to help with my care. Also, as in many families, I am the one with most of the medical skills, so having the http://try.thegrownetwork.com/tiwa/ for them to watch was very useful.

# Seek Treatment for a Venomous Snake Bite Right Away

I am writing my story as an example of how you can be prepared and handle an emergency situation.

But let's be clear:

> *If you get bitten by a snake and you want to try and handle it yourself, you need to have all of the important pieces in place ahead of time.*

Please don't think you can just wing it. The low number of deaths from venomous snakebites is because people seek treatment right away.

I hope this story empowers you to start taking some of those steps.

1. Get to know the possible dangers in your area— what snakes, spiders, or venomous insects share the Earth with you?

2. Start using traditional medicine on small injuries to gain experience and confidence.

3. Work on improving your general health, especially your immune system.

And do you know what the best way to do that is? Start growing your own food!

If you would like to see a short follow-up video a few months after the bite, click on https:// thegrownetwork.com/snake-bite-treatment/.

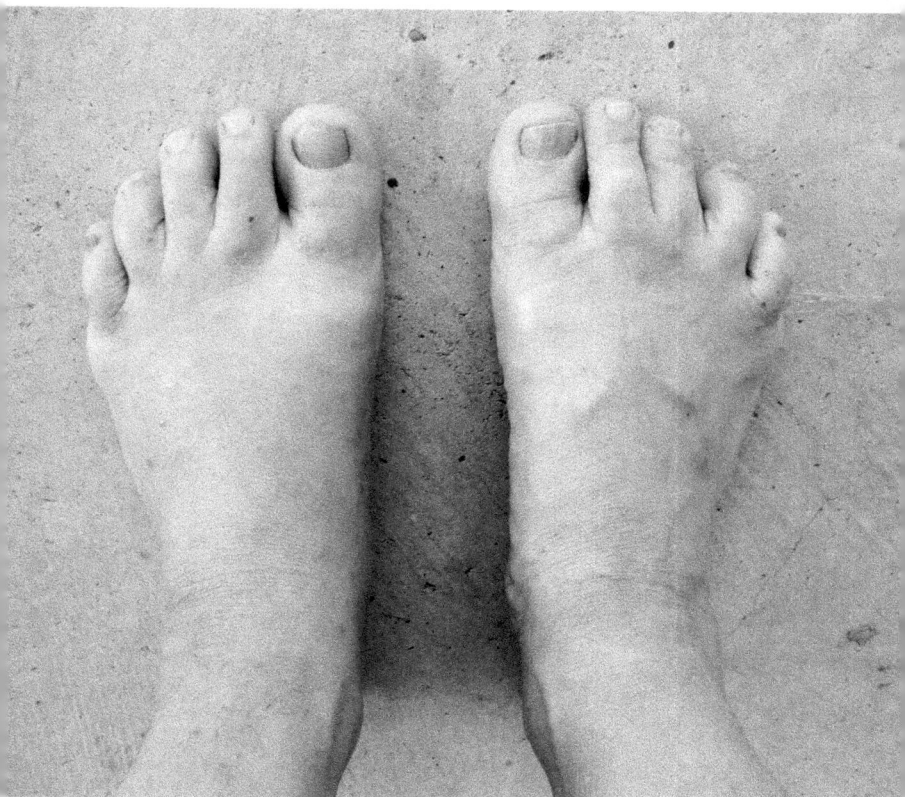

*Snake bite—seven days later all the swelling completely gone*

You can follow Marjory's latest adventures at:

*www.TheGrowNetwork.com*

**Marjory Wildcraft** is the founder of *The Grow Network*, which is the online home of a global community of people who grow their own food and medicine. The purpose of *The Grow Network* is to stop the destruction of the Earth. "Home grown food on every table" is the solution.

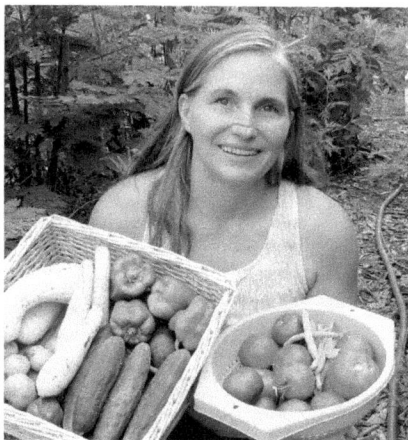

Marjory was featured as an expert in sustainable living by *National Geographic*, she is the host of the *Mother Earth News Online Homesteading Summit*, and is a regular guest on many national radio and television shows. She was recently featured on the cover of *Masters of Health* magazine.

She is an author and producer of several books and videos, but is best known for her DVD series *Grow Your Own Groceries*, which has over a half million copies in use by homesteaders, foodies, preppers, universities, and missionary organizations around the world.